Military Diet

A Strategic Eating Plan for Fast Weight Loss Results

Thomas Rohmer

Copyright © 2018

Disclaimer:

This guide has been created for informational and reference purposes only. The author, publisher, and any other affiliated parties cannot be held in any way accountable for any personal injuries or damage allegedly resulting from the information contained herein, or from any misuse of such guidance. Although strict measures have been taken to provide accurate information, the parties involved with the creation and publication of this guide take no responsibility for any issues that many arise from alleged discrepancies contained herein. It is strongly recommended that you consult a physician, personal trainer, and nutritionist prior to commencing this or any other workout or diet plan. This guide is not a substitute for professional personal guidance from a qualified medical professional. If you feel pain or discomfort at any point during exercises contained herein, cease the activity immediately and seek medical guidance.

Before You Begin:

Get the Latest Scoop on the Most Cutting Edge Info on Health & Fitness!

As thanks for picking up this book, I'd love to offer you the chance to maximize your results by getting exclusive info on health and fitness.

You'll be the first to know when I publish new books, and you'll receive exclusive content on health and fitness that I only share with people on my list.

Simply visit the link directly below and get started on the path to the healthiest version of yourself today!

https://rohmerfitness.lpages.co/kindle-sign-up/

Table of Contents

Chapter 1: What is the Military Diet?.......................7
Chapter 2: How the Military Diet Works..................9
Chapter 3: The Military Diet Meal Plan..................15
Chapter 4: What to Do During the Other Four Days..20
Chapter 5: How to Avoid Rebound Weight Gain on the Military Diet....................................25
Chapter 6: The Military Diet Isn't Just About Eating—You Need to Exercise Too......................33
Chapter 7: Military Diet Mindset.........................43
Chapter 8: Frequently Asked Questions................51

Introduction:

Weight loss is something that a lot of people struggle with considering the fact that 2/3s of the U.S. population is either overweight or obese (1). Why is that? It's not because people are lazy or that they don't care about losing weight.

No, not at all. Instead, it has a lot to do with the fact that people get bored. If I told you that in order to get to a healthy weight all you had to do was eat chicken breast and broccoli for the rest of your life, would you be able to do it?

Maybe for a short time, but after a while you'd get sick and tired of eating the same thing in order to get results. This happens all of the time.

People go on a weight loss diet, only to quit shortly after because the diet was either too hard to keep up with or it was boring. Luckily the military diet will be able to solve that issue for you.

The military diet works in short bursts, allowing you to obtain quick results. Who doesn't want that? However, the problem for most people occurs with what to do afterward.

Yes, it's one thing to lose a bunch of weight in a short period of time, but what are you supposed to do afterward? That's an important question, and that's why I've dedicated an entire chapter to answer that question alone.

You see I don't want you to just have initial success. I want you to achieve success and not have to ever worry about losing it. And the military diet is the perfect diet to be able to help you do just that! Let's jump in and get started...

Chapter 1: What is the Military Diet?

The military diet is a weight loss plan. It's specifically designed to be able to help you lose 10 pounds in 3-7 days.

Of course, you may not lose exactly 10 pounds, but the point is that you're going to lose a good amount of weight in a short period of time. This is something that I really like. You need to be excited about any diet that you're about to start.

If you're about to start a bland diet and you're not sure how long it's going to take you to get results, are you going to be excited about starting that diet? Probably not. As humans, we need targets that we can see and that we know we can hit.

That's the great thing about the military diet. The target is close enough to where we can see it (one week) and that means you'll be more motivated to stick to the actual plan especially since you know the reward that's at the end.

Essentially what you'll be doing on the military diet is following a specific meal plan during the first 3 days, and then during the next 4 days you have some more freedom as to what you can do. I'll discuss what to do during the remaining 4 days of the week in another chapter.

But for now, the main thing you need to know is that you must follow the meal plan during the 3 days. You must also understand how to transition from the 3-day period to the 4-day period, and beyond.

If you mess this up, then you're likely not going to get the results you intended to. But before we get into the specific ins and outs of how the military diet works, it's first important to understand how your body works in regards to burning fat.

Chapter 2: How the Military Diet Works

Most people have a wrong understanding of how their body works in regards to losing weight. People falsely believe that what you eat is the *only* thing that matters when it comes to weight loss.

Their line of thinking is that if you eat healthy, weight loss is guaranteed. If you don't eat healthy then you can forget about having any chance of losing weight, or so their thinking goes.

And I can't blame people for thinking this way. This line of thought has been beaten into our heads that the most important thing for weight loss is what you eat.

I'm here to tell you that's not at all how the body works in regards to weight loss. How much you eat is what matters for weight loss.

You see, the only way your body loses weight is by being in a caloric deficit. A caloric deficit is when you burn off more calories than you consume.

For example, let's say you burn off 2,000 calories in a day. This means that if you eat less than 2,000 calories, you'll start to lose weight.

You must be careful with calories because the reverse is also true. If you eat more calories than you burn off, then you'll start to gain weight.

Using the same example, if you eat more than 2,000 calories, you'll start to gain weight. This is what's known as a caloric surplus.

Since the caloric deficit is the only way your body loses weight, why then is so much emphasis placed on what you eat not how much you eat? Again I think this mentally has been beaten into our heads by supplement and diet companies trying to promote their products.

It simply isn't true. Well, it's not the whole truth I should say. What you eat does matter, but only in the context of how much you're eating.

People assume that it's impossible to overeat healthy foods, but you certainly can. Think about how many calories are contained in foods such as avocados and oatmeal.

It's not far-fetched to think that someone could overeat on calories by consuming these foods. The reason why what you eat matters is because of nutrients.

For example, let's say you eat 100 calories worth of vegetables and I eat 100 calories worth of candy. From a calorie viewpoint, we're equal.

However, the quality of those calories differs greatly. The vegetables you ate contain fiber and other key nutrients that'll help to keep you fuller for a longer period of time.

The candy I ate contains a lot of empty calories and sugar. It'll provide me with no nutritional value, and it'll spike my insulin.

With my insulin levels now being on a roller coaster ride, it could crash at any point, which would leave me feeling hungry again.

So an hour from now, I might have to go back to the kitchen to eat some more food whereas you'll still be good. So yes, what you eat does matter, but if you're not tracking the total amount of calories you're eating, then you're just guessing and hoping that you're eating the right amount.

The best approach is to know how many calories you need to eat (more on this later), track those calories, and then use those calories wisely with the foods you eat. For example, if you need to eat 1,500 calories a day to lose weight, do you think it would be wise to eat nothing but pastries and other junk food? No not at all!

Even though you'd still lose weight, you'd constantly be battling hunger and reckless blood sugar levels. The smarter approach would be to use those calories wisely and eat nutritious filling foods.

This isn't to say that you could never eat junk food because I don't think that approach is good for the long-term either. There needs to be the correct balance.

In fact, the military diet has you eating and drinking specific things for a reason. I'll discuss this more in depth later on, but the main thing I want you to understand is the role that calorie quantity and calorie quality each play in regards to weight loss.

How to Determine the Number of Calories You Need to Eat per Day

The military diet will actually determine how many calories you're going to be eating during the first three days of the diet. There's nothing to have to worry about during those first three days, you simply eat what it tells you to and move on.

However, for the remaining four days of the diet, you'll need to know how many calories you should be eating. You'll also need to measure your calories to ensure you're eating the right amount, which I'll share with you how to do shortly.

First, here's what you need to do to determine how many calories you're burning off in a day. This is also known as your resting metabolic rate, and it's quite easy to calculate.

Simply take your bodyweight, multiply it by 13, and bingo that's your resting metabolic rate. Let's use myself as an example:

Bodyweight 205 x 13=2,665

This means that I burn off 2,665 calories each and every day.

- If I eat more than 2,665 calories per day, I'll be in a caloric surplus, and I'll start to gain weight.
- If I eat less than 2,665 calories per day, I'll be in a caloric deficit, and I'll start to lose weight.
- If I eat right at 2,665 calories per day, I'll be at maintenance, and I'll neither gain nor lose weight.

During the first three days of the military diet, you'll be consuming around 1,100-1,400 calories per day. That's certainly low enough to put most people into a caloric deficit, and if it's not then you probably don't need to be losing weight anyway.

It's after the week is over that you'll still want to know your resting metabolic rate. In my case, I'll want to make sure that I'm still eating less than 2,665 calories. This way I'll still be in a caloric deficit, and I'll still keep on losing weight.

How to Keep Track of Your Calories?

Even if you know how many calories you should be eating on a daily basis, that doesn't do you much good if you have no way of knowing how to track and measure the calories you're eating. That's why you must count your calories.

Yes, I know this can be a real pain, but thanks to technology, it's not that bad. The good news is that you don't have to worry about tracking anything during the first 3 days of the military diet because those calories will already be calculated for you.

However, for everything else you'll be eating outside of those 3 days, you'll want to make sure that you're counting and measuring those calories. Simply put, the best way to do this is to go to the app store and download a calorie counting app.

Some of the apps are free, and some of them are paid. However, don't be afraid to pay a couple of dollars for a solid app.

Most of them will allow you to type in the food that you're eating, and it'll tell you exactly how many calories it contains. Some of them even contain barcode scanners so you can simply scan the barcode label and it'll automatically track the information for you.

Another item you'll want to invest in is a food scale. This'll tell you how many grams your food weighs.

The reason this is important is because you also need to know how much of a certain food you're eating. There's a big difference in calories between 1 cup of oatmeal and 2 cups.

So just make sure that you have a way to accurately measure how much food it is you're eating. Of course you might be wondering, "How do I track calories when I'm eating at a restaurant or some other social event?"

It certainly is harder to measure your calories when you're eating away from home. The best thing you can do is simply take your best guess.

You'll still know what it is that you're eating, so you can still record that in the app. The thing you probably won't know when you're eating at a restaurant is how much of that food you ate.

This is where you'll simply have to use the eyeball test. You'll eyeball how much you ate of a certain food item and log it.

Always ease on the side of estimating eating more and not less. It'd be better to overestimate and still lose weight rather than to underestimate how much you ate and end up not losing any weight.

After a while, you'll get a better sense of how you need to eat in order to lose weight and you can use the eyeball test more often. However, that will only come with time.

Initially, you'll want to be very strict in how you measure and count your calories. Many people simply don't realize how much they've been eating until they start to measure it.

Chapter 3: The Military Diet Meal Plan

The cool thing about the military diet is that there's not a lot of planning involved. I'm going to share with you exactly what you should eat for breakfast, lunch, and dinner during the first 3 days of the diet.

These aren't super expensive or hard to find foods either. In fact, you probably already have most of them in your kitchen right now!

Even if you don't, it won't be much of a hassle because the grocery list for this diet isn't that big. With that being said, here are the first 3 days of what you'll be eating on the military diet:

Day 1: Total Calories approximately 1,400

Breakfast:

- Half a grapefruit
- 1 slice of whole-wheat toast with 2 tablespoons of peanut butter
- 1 cup of black coffee or tea

Lunch:

- Half a cup of tuna
- 1 slice of whole-wheat toast
- 1 cup of black coffee or tea

Dinner:

- 3-oz serving of your choice of meat
- Half a banana
- 1 small apple
- One cup of vanilla ice cream

Day 2: Total Calories approximately 1,200

Breakfast:

- 1 slice of whole-wheat toast
- One egg cooked however you like
- Half a banana
- 1 cup of black coffee or tea

Lunch:

- One egg cooked how you like
- 1 cup of cottage cheese
- 5 saltine crackers
- 1 cup of black coffee or tea

Dinner:

- Two hot dogs with no bun
- ½ cup of broccoli
- ½ cup of carrots
- Half a banana
- Half a cup of vanilla ice cream

Day 3: Total calories approximately 1,100

Breakfast:

- A 1-oz slice of cheddar cheese
- 1 small apple
- 5 saltine crackers

- 1 cup of black coffee or tea

Lunch:

- 1 slice of whole-wheat toast
- 1 egg cooked however you like
- 1 cup of black coffee or tea

Dinner:

- 1 cup of tuna
- Half a banana
- 1 cup of vanilla ice cream

That's all there is to the first 3 days of the diet. Simply eat those foods in the amounts listed. You can eat during the times when you normally eat breakfast, lunch, and dinner. Also, make sure that you drink plenty of water during this time as well.

Why You're Eating the Foods that You Are on the Military Diet

You might be thinking that this is a random combination of foods that you're eating on the military diet. There's actually a method to the madness.

Grapefruit: grapefruit has been shown to help to boost metabolism (2). Therefore it's a great way to start off day 1 of the diet. The faster you can rev up your metabolism, the more weight you're going to lose on this diet.

Black coffee and Tea: you probably noticed that during breakfast and lunch you're going to drink one cup of black coffee or tea. Why is that?

It's because black coffee and tea have been shown to boost metabolism (3). This is similar to the reason why you're eating the grapefruit right off the bat, the goal is to do anything we can to increase our metabolism.

Doing something as small as eating grapefruit or drinking black coffee seems to be a small price to pay for that. Additionally though, black coffee and tea can also help to suppress your appetite.

Since you're going to be eating fewer calories than you usually do, you might get hungry during the day. The black coffee will help you be able to get rid of some of that hunger, which will make it easier to stick to the diet.

Cottage cheese: I remember the first time I ate cottage cheese, I was grossed out by it! The texture and look were so weird to me that I struggled to eat it.

However, now it's one of my favorite foods, and it should be one of yours as well. Once you get over how cottage cheese looks, the taste of it really isn't that bad.

This food is a protein powerhouse containing an average of 14 grams of protein per serving. Not only that, but it contains no carbs and it can be low in fat as well.

The main thing about the protein is that cottage cheese contains a casein protein. This is a protein that's a slower and steadier releasing type of protein.

This way when you eat the cottage cheese, your body won't absorb all of the protein right away. Instead, it'll steadily digest and absorb it throughout the day.

This is important because you want to maximize the protein that you're eating because your calories are being restricted.

Fruits and vegetables: we all know that we should be consuming more fruits and vegetables in our diets, yet many of us struggle to do so. The military diet fortunately contains a fair amount of fruits and vegetables during this 3-day period.

Fruits and vegetables are great because they contain a low amount of calories, but they still contain a high amount of nutrients. These nutrients are key to giving your body the nutrition that it craves, and it'll also help you stay fuller for a longer period of time.

Ice cream: As I mentioned earlier, only eating healthy foods is a recipe for disaster. Who do you know that's been able to start a new diet eating nothing but healthy foods and stick with it for a long period of time?

My guess is probably no one! Or at least no one who was willing to admit that they cheated on their diet!

We all crave sugary and salty foods, and eating some junk food from time to time will help us to keep our sanity. Eating unhealthy foods is how you can make a diet plan sustainable for a long time to come, which is the entire point.

This military diet will do you no good if you lose 10 pounds but then gain it back the following week. Yes ice cream may be unhealthy, but it's all part of the bigger plan.

Chapter 4: What to Do During the Other Four Days

The military diet plan is simple enough during the first 3 days of the diet—simply eat what the meal plan tells you to. However, the other 4 days aren't quite as strict.

In fact, there are no restrictions on what you can and can't eat during the remaining 4 days of the diet plan. It's recommended that you still keep your overall caloric intake low—around 1,500 calories a day.

Therefore during this time, you'll want to make sure that you're still tracking your calories to make sure that you hit your target number. It's also important that you stick to it and not give up after 3 days.

Remember dieting for 3 days is only going to get you so far. Think of the initial 3 days like a jumpstarter.

However, that jumpstarter won't last you forever, and you're going to need a game plan beyond those initial 3 days. That's why it's important to still track your calories and not just go back to the way you were eating before you started the diet.

How Should You Structure Your Eating?

During the first 3 days of the military diet, you eat a standard breakfast, lunch, and dinner with no snacks in between meals. However, during the 4-day part of the diet, you have the freedom to eat however many meals you like.

You can eat one meal per day, six meals per day, the standard 3 meals per day, or whatever else you like. Research has shown that meal frequency doesn't matter for weight loss (4).

There's a myth that it's better to eat smaller meals more frequently because this will help to boost your metabolism, however this simply isn't the case according to the research. Therefore, feel free to eat as frequently or infrequently as you like.

Do whatever it is that works best for you. Personally, I like eating 3 meals per day because it allows me to spend less time preparing and eating food.

It's also important to note that it doesn't matter how many calories you eat per meal. For example, if you're eating 1,500 calories a day across 3 meals, you don't have to eat 500 calories per meal.

If you like eating smaller breakfasts and larger dinners, then you could eat a 250-calorie breakfast and a 750-calorie dinner. Or you could skip breakfast all together and eat a 500-calorie lunch and a 1,000-calorie dinner. You can break it up however it is that you like.

What Should You Eat During This Part of the Diet?

Another big question is what should I eat during the last 4 days? The thing is there are no limits to what you can and can't eat during this part of the diet.

That may be a good thing or a bad thing depending on how you look at it! Remember from chapter 2, the first thing you want to worry about is calorie quantity.

In this case, you'll want to make sure that you set your boundaries to 1,500 calories per day. That'll then help you be able to set up which foods you'll eat and in what amounts.

Now I'm not going to be able to tell you exactly what to eat every day for the rest of your life. In fact, that would only hinder you, not help you.

Imagine if I tried to give you a meal plan for every day of your life. It would cripple you because you wouldn't know how to adapt to situations that you'd find yourself in.

For example, let's say a meal plan tells you that you should be eating chicken, brown rice, and broccoli for a meal. However, you're at a party and none of those food items are there.

What do you do? You get stuck and paralyzed because you don't know what you should eat at the party! However, if instead you understood the basic principles of weight loss (which you should by now), then you'll know what to do.

You could say, "Ok I know I'm going to a party tomorrow night. Therefore I'll eat fewer calories than I normally do during the day so I can enjoy myself at the party.

I'll save enough calories to where I can enjoy an 800-calorie meal at the party. This way I'll still hit my caloric target and be able to continue losing weight."

My philosophy is that it's better to teach a man how to fish rather than to give a man a fish. However, if you're still not sure how often you should be eating healthy versus not healthy, then this might help you out...

Follow the Golden Rule

Ok so when you're not following the first 3 days of the military diet, how often should you eat junk food? As I talked about earlier, eating too much junk food can be dangerous because it can cause crashes in your blood sugar levels, which will make your hungry at random times.

Having to fight these food cravings all day long is a recipe for disaster, and it'll only cause you to eat more in the long run. Therefore, it isn't a good idea to eat however you please even if you're eating the correct amount of calories to still be able to lose weight.

On the flip side though, you don't want to completely eliminate junk food because then you'll go insane and likely quit on your diet plan. That's why you need to have a balance.

The best way I've found to do this is to follow my golden rule of eating clean healthy foods roughly 85% of the time and eating junk food the remaining 15%. This way you're still eating healthy foods the majority of the time, and getting the benefits from eating nutrient-rich foods.

Additionally, you're still able to satisfy any cravings that you may have, which will make it easier for you to be able to stick to the nutrition plan. You can break up this 15% however it is that you like.

You could save it up and have a day where you can eat whatever foods you like. Or you can have a little treat every day like a small bowl of ice cream.

What to Do If You Want More Structure

If you want more structure for how you should be eating during this part of the nutrition plan, then you can follow a similar outline to how you ate during the first 3 days of the diet. So this would mean doing things like drinking black coffee or tea for breakfast and lunch.

It would also mean consuming fruits and/or vegetables with most of your meals. And finally, it would also entail being able to enjoy yourself from time to time by eating a small bowl of ice cream etc.

The cool thing is that you'll get to add in some more calories because during this 4-day period you're allowed to eat 1,500 calories per day instead of 1,100-1,400. You can add in these extra calories however it is that you like.

This could mean eating some extra fruit or maybe an extra egg or two during lunch. You can mix and match it however you like, but this is just a simple way to add in some structure if you really have no idea how you should eat, and you're afraid that you'll mess things up.

Chapter 5: How to Avoid Rebound Weight Gain on the Military Diet

The last thing you want to happen is to lose a bunch of weight quickly but then quickly gain it all back in a short period of time. That's where a real issue could arise with the military diet.

The diet only lasts for a week, but then what are you supposed to do after that initial week is up? This chapter will help you to be able to answer that question.

What Usually Happens on a Typical Diet

Here's what usually happens to most people who want to lose weight and try to do so by dieting. Let's use an example of a made-up person named Joe:

- Step 1: Joe decides that he wants to lose weight.
- Step 2: Joe eliminates all unhealthy food out of his diet.
- Step 3: for the first-week things are going smoothly and Joe has even lost some weight.
- Step 4: Joe gets tempted at work when lunch gets catered or he doesn't feel like cooking and gets some fast food.
- Step 5: Joe feels as if he completely ruined his diet, so he says "forget this" and proceeds to binge eat everything he can.
- Step 6: Joe returns to his normal way eating and gains all of the weight back he lost plus a little bit more.

- Step 7: After a couple weeks when Joe's feeling better about himself and confident that he'll surely lose weight this time, he starts a new diet and the process starts itself over again.

This is a trap that I've seen so many people fall into who desperately want to lose weight. There's nothing wrong with wanting to get some quick results to help keep you motivated, but you also have to think of the long-term game.

That's why so many people fail to keep the weight off. Putting yourself through mistery to lose weight is one thing, but having to continue in that misery is a nightmare you can only bare so long.

That's why you must make the military diet a sustainable approach. There's a reason why the first part of the diet only lasts for 3 days and then the next part is more flexible.

The reason is because you won't be able to stick to that initial 3-day plan for much longer than 3 days. Imagine only being able to eat 1,100 calories every day for the rest of your life.

Do you really think you'd be able to maintain that? My guess is probably not.

That's why it's so important to vary things so that you're still losing weight, but at the same time still be able to keep your sanity. Here's what I mean—for the first week of the diet follow it as is.

Meaning you'll follow the meal plan and eat roughly 1,100-1,400 calories during the first 3 days of the diet. Then during the next 4 days of the plan, eat how you like, but make sure that you don't exceed 1,500 calories per day.

After the first week is up, you'll want to change things accordingly based on how you're feeling. The cool thing about the military diet is that it only lasts for a week, and you can even change up how you do the 4-day period.

This means that you can easily do the military diet during one week out of the month, every six weeks, or something similar. Doing the military diet every week might be too strenuous and hard to keep up with.

So instead you can give yourself breaks by following the military diet every 2-12 weeks depending on how much weight you want to lose and how fast you want to lose it. Let's say you follow the military diet, and after a week you lost 10 pounds.

This is a great start, but you're probably going to want to lose more weight than 10 pounds. If that's the case, I'd recommend waiting before you try to dive right back into another military diet.

Go ahead and during the next week, eat more calories, but not too much to where you're not in a caloric deficit anymore. Using myself as an example, my resting metabolic rate was determined to be 2,665 calories in chapter 2 by multiplying my bodyweight by 13.

This means that I'll want to eat less than 2,665 calories a day so that I can keep losing weight. Since I just finished eating a low amount of calories the previous week, the following week I could allow myself to eat more calories such as 2,100-2,200 for example.

This way I'll still be in a caloric deficit so I'll still be able to continue losing weight, but I'll also be able to enjoy myself more because I'll get to eat more calories. This is what will make the approach more sustainable.

The week after that, I could even eat at maintenance calories (2,665 in my case). I won't be losing any weight this week, however I could use this week to help prepare myself for the following week where I might go for another military diet.

I could even do a partial military diet where I only follow the initial 3-day eating plan and then go back to eating at maintenance calories. The main point is that you don't want to continuously follow the military diet week after week after week because you're going to crash and burn.

This diet is meant to be done in short bursts. The initial 3-day period can be tough, but after that, it gets a little bit easier. The 4-day period that follows can be tough as well, but once the week is up you can add in more calories during the next week if you like.

What you want to avoid is going back to eating the way you used to if that entailed not tracking your calories and eating what you wanted when you wanted. The problem with going back to your normal eating patterns is that you'll likely overeat and gain some of the weight back that you worked so hard to lose.

That's why no matter what, even if it's an off week from the military diet, you still need to have a caloric intake goal in mind and track your calories to make sure you're not going above that number. I understand that it can be enticing to try and lose all of the weight rapidly, but think about sustainability here.

I want you to lose the weight and not have to worry about it coming back. There's no specific pattern to how you should go about things, judge it based on how you feel.

If at the start of a week you feel really run down and irritable, then maybe eating more calories at maintenance level or a slight deficit would be best. If on the other hand, you're feeling good and that you can push yourself to create a larger deficit, then by all means go for it.

There's no right or wrong way to go about it. You have to do what's in your best interest to make this approach last for a long time to come. Here's an idea of how you could do things using myself as an example:

- Week 1: follow the military diet (1,100-1,400 calories for 3 days and 1,500 calories for 4 days)
- Week 2: eat at a deficit of 500 calories (2,165 calories per day in my case)
- Week 3: eat at a deficit of 250 calories (2,415 calories per day in my case)
- Week 4: eat at a deficit of 100 calories (2,565 calories per day in my case)
- Week 5: eat at maintenance calories (2,656 calories per day in my case)
- Week 6: follow the military diet again (1,100-1,400 calories for 3 days and 1,500 calories for 4 days)

Note: you can extend things out for as long or as little as you feel like. If you want to do the military diet every 4 weeks, then you could shorten it by eating in a deficit of 500 calories the week after the military diet, a caloric deficit of 250 calories the next week, and then the military diet the week after that.

Or if you'd rather do 8 or 12 weeks, you certainly can. You could do something like eat in a 500 calorie deficit for 2 weeks, then a 250 calorie deficit for the following 2 weeks, and so on and so forth until you're ready to start your next military diet.

You'll notice in the example that I'm increasing my caloric intake from week-to-week and it's for a good reason. Doing things in this manner will help you work with your body's hormones and it'll help to prevent some rebound weight gain.

Your body has a hormone called leptin. Basically, it's a hormone that regulates fat storage.

When you restrict your calories, leptin levels decrease, which causes you to want to eat more and burn less fat. On the flip side, when we eat more calories, leptin levels increase, which causes us to eat less and burn more fat.

What it boils down to is that leptin tells our brains how much fat is stored in our cells, and I'm sure you can see the paradox that exists with this hormone.

In order to lose weight, you must eat fewer calories. However, when you do that, your leptin levels will decrease.

When you have decreased leptin levels in your body, you'll be stimulated to eat more, which in turn will cause you to not burn more fat. This is definitely an issue you'd run into if you kept on going with the military diet week after week.

You'd run your leptin levels into the ground, and it'd only be a matter of time before you can't take it anymore. Therefore, by tapering our calories upwards in the weeks following the military diet, you'll be able to steadily increase your leptin levels and avoid a big-time crash.

Then once your leptin levels are back to normal, you can do the military diet again, lose more weight, and repeat the process. This is the smartest way to go about things so that you don't constantly have to fight your body's hormones. Of course, you don't have to approach things in this manner, but it makes the nutrition plan way easier to sustain for a long period of time.

What Should I Eat During Weeks that I'm Not Following the Military Diet?

Right now you might be wondering how it is that you should eat during the weeks when you're not doing the military diet. You have the freedom to eat how you like during these weeks.

The main thing you want to focus on is making sure that you're eating the correct amount of calories. If you eat too much, you'll end up gaining weight and ruining your progress.

Then you'll want to focus on what it is that you're going to eat. I'd recommend following a similar plan that you would follow during the 4-day phase of the military diet, with the exception that you'll get to consume more calories.

So do things like eating healthy 85% of the time with foods like fruits, vegetables, whole grains, and lean meats. Eat your favorite foods the other 15% of the time.

Eat as frequently or infrequently as you need to in a way that fits best with your schedule. If you know that you're going to go to a social event, be smart and plan ahead.

Save some of your calories for later so that you can actually enjoy yourself at the event. Doing things like this will allow you to make great strides in your weight loss journey and be able to keep the weight off for good.

Think of this military diet strategy like high-intensity interval training. In case you're unfamiliar, high-intensity interval training is a form of cardio where you alternate between a high intensity and a low intensity.

So for example, on a treadmill, you might alternate between running at a speed of 8 mph for 30 seconds and walking at a speed of 3 mph for 30 seconds. That's very similar to what you'd be doing with this long-term military diet approach.

You're essentially going to be alternating between periods of greater weight loss and periods of lesser weight loss. For example, during the week that you're doing the military diet, you could lose up to 10 pounds.

Then on the following weeks, when you're increasing your calories, you're not going to lose as much weight, however those extra calories are going to allow you to be able to push yourself hard again when it's time to do another week of the military diet.

Similarly, when doing high-intensity interval training, the lower intensity cardio (such as the walking in this case) will allow you to recuperate and be able to give your best effort during the higher intensity phase of the intervals.

On the surface level, it might make more sense to just go week after week after week doing the military diet. But think about this—would it make sense to get on a treadmill and do an all-out sprint for 20 minutes? No of course not!

You would get tired and slow down, you wouldn't be able to do a max sprint for 20 minutes! It would make way more sense to sprint for a shorter period of time that you could handle, and wait to sprint again until you've fully recuperated.

It's the same way with the military diet. The weeks following the military diet will allow your body to be able to recuperate and help to prepare you for the next time you do the military diet.

Chapter 6: The Military Diet Isn't Just About Eating—You Need Exercise Too

When you think of someone in the military, what do you think of? You probably think of someone who's tough, fit, and willing to take on any challenge necessary to get the job done.

You probably don't think of someone who solely focuses on their nutrition. And that's why training is also necessary.

These soldiers aren't just worried about what they eat; they're also concerned with their fitness level. You definitely don't want to go into combat being out of shape, you need to be ready for anything!

And training your body with exercise is the best way to go about doing that. Even if you're not an athlete or in the military, exercise will still provide you with many health benefits.

Think about the things you do on a regular or semi-regular basis such as walking up stairs, unloading groceries, gardening, helping a friend move, etc. These are the kinds of things that exercise can help you get in shape and be prepared for.

You won't have to worry about getting completely gassed going up one flight of stairs. The research is clear on the health benefits that exercise will provide you with such as lowering your risk for diseases such as cardiovascular disease among others (5).

Exercise will also help with depression, make you feel more energized, and help you live a longer life (6). Additionally, exercise will also give you some more leeway in your nutrition plan.

This will either allow you to lose weight even faster, or it'll allow you to be able to eat more food while still being able to lose weight. For example, if you do a workout and burn 300 calories, then you could eat 300 more calories worth of food for the day and still be ok.

Or you could eat the same amount of food that you normally would and create an even bigger caloric deficit. Finally, you could even mix it up however you like. For example, if you did a workout and burned 300 calories, you could eat an additional 200 calories and still have created a caloric deficit that's 100 calories more than if you hadn't exercised at all.

Not only that, but exercise will help you be able to build your best body possible. You may or may not be interested in training to build a better-looking body, but exercising certainly won't hurt anything.

If you think about it, adding in an exercise routine makes total sense. The military diet is great because it can help you lose weight quickly, which if you had a short period of time to prepare for combat, then this nutrition plan is great. But there's also another side that exists.

You also need to be physically fit for combat, and much the same way with the diet plan, there are different things you can do to shorten the amount of time it takes to get in shape physically. Of course, you don't have to follow any exercise plan when doing the military diet.

The choice is ultimately yours to make as to what you want to do. In case you do want to exercise so you can have a complete routine, I'm going to share with you some of the things that you can do for exercise.

Resistance Training

Weight lifting is great for many reasons. It'll help you build more muscle, prevent osteoporosis, and help you burn fat. It'll also help you tone and firm up your muscles, which is something that diet alone can't do for you.

If all you use to lose weight is your diet, then you'll end up looking flat and weak when you reach your goal bodyweight. However, if you lift weights and diet, then you'll look fit and firm.

Resistance training is great for both men and women. Many women are afraid to lift weights because they fear that it might make them look bulky.

This isn't true. Women who regularly lift weights have the fittest bodies. The reality of the matter is that women produce about 10% of the testosterone that men do (7).

Testosterone is a hormone that's responsible for fat distribution, bone mass, and muscle and strength, among other things. That's why a man is bigger, stronger, faster, and leaner than a woman on average.

That should be relieving if you're a woman who's hesitant about lifting weights. Your body simply won't allow you to become as big as a man unless of course, you get aid from something like drugs.

However, if you're a natural lifter, you have nothing to worry about, and lifting weights as a female will only benefit your health and how you look, not hinder it. With that being said, here are a couple of different weight lifting routines that you can follow if you're interested in starting a resistance training routine:

The first workout routine you can do consists of 3 full-body weight workouts per week. You'll complete the same workout every time you go to the gym. You can set up your workout schedule in one of the following ways:

- Monday: Workout
- Tuesday: Rest
- Wednesday: Workout
- Thursday: Rest
- Friday: Workout
- Saturday: Rest
- Sunday: Rest

Or

- Monday: Rest
- Tuesday: Workout
- Wednesday: Rest
- Thursday: Rest
- Friday: Rest
- Saturday: Rest
- Sunday: Rest

Full-body workouts will provide you with many benefits:

- You'll burn more calories from your workouts.
- You'll gain strength and muscle faster since you'll be stimulating your muscles more frequently.
- You'll have better nervous system recovery because you won't train on consecutive days.
- You'll develop the perfect form on key lifts faster because you practice them more often.

Essentially your body has never been exposed to this stimulus (i.e. weightlifting) before. Therefore, you can take advantage of what some people call "beginner gains." And by increasing the frequency at which you stimulate your muscle groups, you can speed up the process.

Side Note: A set is a group of consecutive repetitions. A repetition is one complete motion of an exercise. And the rest period is how long of a break you'll take until you start the next set. For example, let's say you're completing, sets of 8 reps and resting 2 minutes in between sets for the barbell squat exercise.

You'll squat down and stand back up, completing the movement of the exercise and one rep. You'll repeat that motion 7 more times for a total of 8 repetitions. That will complete the set and you will begin your rest period. Once your 2-minute rest period is up, you'll start the next set and perform another 8 repetitions.

That will complete set number 2, and you'll rest another 2 minutes. Once that time period is up, you'll complete the final set of 8 repetitions, and then you'll move onto the next exercise.

Here's the workout:

- Incline Dumbbell Bench Press: 3 sets 8 reps 2 min rest between (btw) sets
- Barbell Back Squats: 3 sets of 8 reps 2 min rest btw sets
- Lat Pulldowns: 3 sets of 10 reps 90 sec rest btw sets
- Standing DB Military Press: 3 sets of 8 reps 2 min rest btw sets
- Seated DB Curls: 3 sets of 12 reps 60 sec rest btw sets
- Tricep Straight Bar Pushdowns: 3 sets of 12 reps 60 sec rest btw sets

That's all there is to it! Don't let the simplicity of it fool you—it will work.

Here's a different workout routine you can do if you don't want to work all of the muscles in your body during one workout:

This workout contains 4 workouts per week. It contains 2 different workouts—A and B. You'll alternate between workout A and B every time you go to the gym. Set up your gym schedule in 1 of the following 2 ways:

- Monday: Workout A
- Tuesday: Workout B
- Wednesday: Rest Day
- Thursday: Workout A
- Friday: Workout B
- Saturday: Rest Day
- Sunday: Rest Day

Or

- Monday: Workout A
- Tuesday: Workout B
- Wednesday: Rest Day
- Thursday: Workout A
- Friday: Rest Day
- Saturday: Workout B
- Sunday: Off

The second option will give you an extra day of rest in between workouts, which will help with central nervous system recovery. Feel free to pick whatever best fits your schedule.

Workout A: Chest, Shoulders, and Triceps

- Incline Barbell or Dumbbell Bench Press: 3 sets of 6 reps 3 min rest btw sets
- Standing Dumbbell Military Press: 3 sets of 6 reps 3 min rest btw sets
- Dumbbell Skull Crushers: 3 sets of 8 reps 90 sec rest btw sets
- Standing Dumbbell Lateral Raises: 3 sets of 10-12 reps 60 sec rest btw sets
- Bent Lateral Raises: 3 sets of 10-12 reps 60 sec rest btw sets

Workout B: Back, Biceps, and Legs

- Weighted Pull-Ups (replace with lat pulldowns if you're unable to do pull-ups): 3 sets of 6 reps 3 min rest btw sets
- Standing Dumbbell Curls: 3 sets of 8 reps 90 sec rest btw sets
- Bulgarian Split Squats: 3 sets of 8 reps (per leg) 2 min rest btw sets
- Bent Over Row: 3 sets of 8 reps 2 min rest btw sets
- Hammer Curls: 3 sets of 10-12 reps 60 sec rest btw sets

What to Do for Cardio

Of course, you aren't just limited to lifting weights as your only means of exercise. You can also do cardio.

As I mentioned earlier with resistance training, cardio will be great for burning extra calories to help you reach your goal weight faster or give you some more leeway in your diet plan. Ultimately the best form of cardio is cardio that you'll actually do.

I'll share with you in a bit what the research says is the best form of cardio, however don't feel obligated to do your cardio in this manner. If you find it boring or not your style, then you'll likely never do it on a consistent basis.

And any form of cardio is certainly better than doing nothing at all. With that being said, the best way to do cardio is by combining high-intensity interval training (HIIT) and slow steady state cardio.

As I mentioned earlier, HIIT is a form of cardio where you alternate between a high intensity and a low intensity. Steady state cardio is simply picking one speed (such as 3.5 mph on a treadmill for example) and staying at that same pace for the duration of your cardio workout. Studies has shown higher intensity cardio results in more fat loss over time than lower intensity cardio (8) (9).

HIIT really is efficient—you're burning more calories in less time. HIIT's even cooler though when combined with slow steady state cardio. The reason why is because the HIIT will release free fatty acids into the bloodstream, and then the slow steady state cardio will burn off those free fatty acids.

Most people will do HIIT but won't follow it up with slow steady state cardio. This is a shame because all of those free fatty acids released into the bloodstream will get reabsorbed.

Here's how to do a combo cardio workout:

Note: This cardio workout can be done on any type of cardio machine (treadmill, elliptical, etc.), outside, on a track or wherever else you want. No matter where you are, the workout will be the same.

Combo Cardio Workout

#1: 10-15 minutes of HIIT on a treadmill (or cardio machine of choice)

-Sprint for 30 seconds

-Walk for 1 minute (alternate between sprinting and walking for the full 10-15 min)

#2: Immediately followed by 10-15 minutes of steady state cardio

-Walk on treadmill at 3.5 mph

Now the cool thing about HIIT is that you can adjust it to your current fitness level. For example, if you can't sprint for 30 seconds, do a fast jog for 20 seconds (7.5 mph on a treadmill as an example) and then walk for 1 minute and 10 seconds.

You could even do 45 seconds of sprinting and 45 seconds of walking if you're in better shape. You can customize it to your needs, but you have to do the HIIT first followed by the slow steady state cardio.

I recommend that you do this 20-30 minute workout 2 times per week. I wouldn't advise that you do it any more than 2 times per week because that's too much and it's not necessary beyond that point.

What About Walking?

The thing is high intensity interval training may not be for you. It might be too intense or sometimes you may just want to do a lesser form of cardio. If that's the case for you, then you can most certainly walk. You don't have to completely give up cardio altogether just because you don't feel like doing high intensity interval training.

Walking is great because it can help to reduce stress (10) and speed up recovery from a hard workout. Walking also helps with lymphatic system recovery, and there's research showing how walking more (or moving more in general for that matter) can reduce your risk of developing heart disease (11).

Best of all, walking is an easy way to burn more calories. I used to think that walking was only for people who weren't in that good of shape, but boy was I wrong about that! Walking should be done by everyone, fit or unfit. The simple fact is that walking provides benefits that the higher intensity cardio can't.

I recommend going for walks around town or at the local park. Go outside and get some fresh air. Walking for 30 minutes 3 days a week would be enough to start providing you with some amazing benefits. You can still do the combination cardio workout twice per week in addition to the walking if you want to.

Chapter 7: Military Diet Mindset

Only the strong survive the tough rigors of being in the military. You must be in shape not just physically but mentally as well. And the same goes for the military diet.

In order to be successful with this type of diet, you must be able to have the right mindset and approach in order to be successful. That's why it's important to set goals and know your why or your motivation.

Think about it—most people who go on a diet don't set goals or think about why it is that they want to achieve a certain fitness result. Then when things get tough, they quit because they don't have any motivation to keep on going.

If you want to be successful with your diet plan unlike most people, then you have to be willing to do what they won't. And setting goals and finding your why is a great way to do just that. Whenever things get tough and you feel like quitting, you can look back at your goals and remember why you started down this path in the first place.

How to Properly Set Goals

There's certainly a wrong way and a right way to go about setting your goals. Most people have a vague idea in their heads as to what it is that they want, and they think that's good enough.

For example, you might have a goal of losing 20 pounds, but that goal isn't real until you transfer it from your head to paper. Writing your goals down with pen and paper is what makes your goals real.

Up until that point, they're simply just an idea in your head. Writing your goals down makes it a real thing for your subconscious mind, if not it's just another thought in your head that won't be taken seriously.

Therefore, the first thing you must do when it comes to setting goals is to make sure that you actually write your goals down. Secondly, you'll want to write out your goals in the present tense as if you've already achieved them.

This is going to help set you up for success and start to train your subconscious mind as if you've already got what it is that you want. This is more powerful than you might think.

For example, the next time you're feeling in a bad mood, take note of your posture. You'll probably notice that you're slouched over, with your head down, and your shoulders rounding forward.

Once you've noticed how your posture is, change it by sitting up straight, head up tall, and shoulders back. See how you feel after changing your posture.

You'll notice a difference in your mood because your mind will follow patterns that it sees. Whenever you're out and about, take notice of your posture and make sure you're walking tall with your shoulders back and a smile on your face. You'll notice that when you walk like this, you instantly feel like a more confident person.

So if you write your goals as if you've already achieved them, then your mind will follow suit and start to act as if you've already achieved your goals. It certainly makes a difference.

So don't say something like, "I will weigh 150 pounds by July 10, 2018." Instead say something like, "I weigh 150 pounds by July 10, 2018."

Sure consciously you may know that you don't weigh 150 pounds yet, but writing your goals this way isn't for your conscious mind, it's for your subconscious, which doesn't know the difference.

You probably noticed from the example goal above that there was a date attached to the goal. This is the third step you'll want to take when setting your goals.

Again this is something that of the people who do set goals, many of them don't set a date for when to achieve it by. This is a huge mistake because if there's no date, then there's no sense of urgency for accomplishing it.

You may get around to achieve it one day or maybe you won't—who cares! That's the kind of attitude you're adopting whether you realize it or not when you don't set a date for your goals.

In terms of what timeframes you should use when setting a date, take your best guess for how long you think it'll take you to achieve it. There's no hard rule that you're only allowed a month to set a goal and accomplish it for example.

Some goals will take longer than others in order for you to achieve. And if you set a goal to be achieved by July 10, 2018 for example and you don't hit your target, then simply set a new date to achieve the goal by.

In this case, maybe you fell just short of achieving your goal by July 10th; so instead, you reset the goal date to July 20, 2018. And if you unfortunately don't reach your goal by July 20th, go ahead and set a new date until you hit the goal.

The key to setting dates is to try and find a sweet spot where you're pushing yourself in order to achieve it. If you set the date too far away, then it becomes easy to procrastinate and not even get started until a later date.

Therefore, don't be afraid to set your achievement dates on the earlier side because you can always adjust them later if you need to. It definitely doesn't mean that you're a failure if you don't achieve it by your original date.

After you set a date for your goals, the next thing you'll want to do is post your goals where you can easily see them. It doesn't do you any good to write your goals down, and then hide them as if you want to forget about them.

I keep my goals up in front of my computer so I can easily see them when I'm working. You need to do the same with your goals so that you can constantly be reminded of them and motivated by them.

Aside from the list you'll have in front of you, you'll also want to make sure that you write your goals down every morning and night. This might seem like a pain, but remember **you must do what others won't so you can do what they can't.**

By writing your goals first thing in the morning, you'll be excited by them and they'll be on your mind throughout the day. Then when you write them again before going to bed, they'll be in your subconscious mind throughout the night.

Finally, don't be afraid to set multiple goals and feel free to set goals for other areas of your life besides fitness. You could set relationship goals and financial goals as well. Here are a couple of examples of fitness goals that you could set:

- I weigh 140 pounds by August 20th, 2018.
- I lose 25 pounds by September 5th, 2018.
- I bench press 200 pounds by October 12th, 2018.

- I complete the Military Diet with ease by June 25th, 2018.

These are a few examples, but it should be enough to get your mind churning with ideas.

Process Goals Vs. Outcome Goals

There are two different types of goals—outcome and process goals. The type of goals I mentioned in the previous section such as, "I weigh 140 pounds by August 20th, 2018" are outcome goals.

These goals are great because they're where you want to go. Think of setting goals like a mountain.

Outcome goals are like the top of the mountain because that's the end destination. Without the end destination, you'd have no clue where you're going.

On the other hand, there are also process goals. These are things you're going to do in order to achieve the outcome goal.

Think of process goals like climbing up a mountain. Process goals are what you must do in order to achieve your outcome goals. Here are some examples of outcome goals and how they relate to process goals.

Outcome Goal:

- I weigh 140 pounds by August 20th, 2018.

Process Goals:

- I do a high-intensity interval-training workout 3 times per week.

- I drink at least half my bodyweight in ounces of water per day.
- I follow the Military Diet once a week every six weeks.

It's a good rule of thumb to have more process goals than you do outcome goals. Process goals make up a bigger chunk of the mountain. I usually like to have at least 3 process goals for every 1 outcome goal that I set.

Now you might be wondering, well should I focus more of my attention on outcome or process goals? I say focus on whatever motivates you more.

For most people, that's going to be the outcome goals. Think about it this way—if you're climbing a mountain and you forget about why you're climbing it in the first place, you may very well turn around and go back home.

Most likely you started climbing the mountain because you wanted to get to the top of it! That's why you'll want to keep your eyes set on the prize, to help motivate you to keep on moving forward. Use your process goals like tools to help remind you of what it is that you need to do in order to continue climbing up the mountain.

Don't Just Set Your Goals, Find Your Why

Sure you may want to lose 20 pounds, but why is that? Surely you have a reason for why it is that you want to achieve that certain goal.

Finding your why is another great way to help motivate you to keep on moving forward even when things get tough. And once again, most people have no clue what their why is.

They wonder around aimlessly, and this is why most people fail to lose weight and keep it off. It's not because they're lazy, it's because they don't know how to hone in their attention, focus on one thing, and keep themselves motivated long enough in order to accomplish it.

Therefore, finding your why is very important because the stronger your why is, the more likely it is you're going to get results. Let's say for example you have a goal of weighing 140 pounds. Ask yourself why it is that you want to weigh 140 pounds:

Why do I want to weigh 140 pounds?

- I want to feel more attractive.

This is a good start, but it can go deeper than this. Ask yourself why you want to feel more attractive:

- I want to go on more dates.

Ok now we're starting to get somewhere, but we can still go deeper than this. Ask yourself why one more time to get to the root reason why it is that you want to weigh 140 pounds:

- I want to be in a relationship.

Great! You now know that the real reason why you want to lose weight is because you want to get into a relationship. This isn't something that you need to be ashamed of if this is what's going to excite you and motivate you to get in better shape.

If your why is something like, "I want to get healthy," that may not be exciting enough to get you to take action. That's why you need to ask yourself why 3 times to get to the root of why it is that you want to get in better shape. Let's use another example with the first why being, "I want to get healthy."

Why do you want to get healthy?

- I want to have more energy.

Why do you want to have more energy?

- I want to be able to keep up with my kids all day long.

So the real motivation, in this case, is to get healthy so you can keep up with your kids and be able to play with them for longer periods of time. This is great.

You can write down all three of your original whys (and any others you may have) and keep it next to your other sheet with your goals on them. Then whenever things start to get tough (which they certainly will), you can think about your kids and how much it would mean to them if you were able to accomplish this goal.

Essentially goal setting and finding your why will give you something you can rely on to help you achieve your life aspirations. Most people unfortunately, don't have this sort of system in place, and it makes it a lot harder to achieve what they want.

Chapter 8: Frequently Asked Questions

Can I Repeat the Military Diet Week After Week?

Yes you could repeat the military diet week after week if you really wanted to. However, I don't think that would last very long as a sustainable option for you to lose weight and keep it off.

Instead, I think you're much better off doing the military diet for one week, taking a break where you eat more calories, and then hitting it hard again with the military diet. Of course how often you choose to do the military diet is up to you, but the best way to go about it would be to do the military diet every six weeks.

And each week that leads up to the military diet, you'd increase your caloric intake slightly as I described in chapter five.

I Gained Weight When I Started Eating More Calories. What Should I Do?

This is normal and should be expected, so the best thing you can do is not freak out and stay calm. The reason for this is because your bodyweight will fluctuate.

So when you're eating less calories, your glycogen stores will be lower. However, when you start to eat more calories, your muscles will fill up with more glycogen, which will cause a slight increase in bodyweight because glycogen isn't massless.

Therefore, it's not actual fat that you're gaining here and that's why the number on the scale can be misleading. Don't be fooled by this and think that you always need to push yourself with eating low calories week after week because that'll only lead to burnout.

Instead be patient and realize that most of your weight loss will occur during the weeks when you're following the military diet. With that being the case, you may be tempted to do the military diet week after week, but remember we're seeking long-term sustainability here not quick results.

If you're going to be paranoid by the number on the scale, only weigh yourself once a week first thing in the morning after you use the bathroom. By weighing yourself in a consistent manner such as this, you'll be able to better judge if you've actually lost weight instead of just having to worry if your bodyweight is simply fluctuating.

What if I'm Not Losing Weight at 13 Calories per Pound of Bodyweight?

Let's say you calculate your resting metabolic rate by multiplying your bodyweight by 13. You still follow the military diet as it's laid out, but during the weeks when you're not following the military diet, your weight loss has stalled.

What should you do? The first thing to remember is that this really isn't that big of a deal.

Most of your weight loss should be occurring during the weeks when you're following the military diet. During weeks when you're not following the military diet, you're going to be eating in smaller caloric deficits or even at maintenance so weight loss won't be as great.

However, if you really want to, you can decrease your calories slightly more to help increase weight loss during the weeks when you're not doing the military diet. For example, you could start with 12 calories per pound of bodyweight, and then work your way down to 11 or even 10 calories per pound of bodyweight.

I know it can be tempting to want to cut your calories as low as possible, but once again, you need to remember the long game here. It's better to slow down and follow the military diet in a manner that'll allow you to be able to actually keep the weight off once you lose it.

Do I Have to Exercise in Order to See Results with This Diet?

No, you certainly don't have to exercise in order to start seeing results with the military diet. I included a chapter on exercise so you'd have a plan for what you could do if you were interested, but it's not mandatory by any means.

You will be able to get results just from following the military diet by itself. Exercise will allow you to be able to get results faster or give you more leeway in your diet plan, which is pretty cool. So if you want to experience the benefits of exercise, then by all means do it.

Do I Have to Eat the Specific Foods on the Military Diet?

If you don't eat the foods on the military diet that it tells you to eat, then you're not really following the military diet. The foods you eat on the diet are chosen for a reason, and therefore it's best if you follow it as it's laid out.

However, there's nothing binding you to eating those specific foods if you absolutely don't want to or can't. You could make modifications here and there if you absolutely had too, and you'd still be able to get results as long as you're in a caloric deficit.

Therefore, with any changes you decide to make, be sure you're still staying at roughly the same amount of calories. If you make changes that cause you to overeat, then you won't lose any weight.

Should I Focus More On Cardio or Weights if I Do Decide to Exercise?

You can do whatever you enjoy more because that's what will make you more likely to exercise in the first place. You can also do both weight lifting and cardio if you'd like.

The main thing here is to consider what you want to get out of exercise. If you just want to burn some extra calories, get your heart rate up, and/or improve your conditioning, then cardio will get the job done.

On the other hand, if you want to firm up your muscles or even build muscle, then you'll want to lift weights. Lifting weights will still be a great way to burn calories as well to aid in weight loss.

Are There Any Supplements that I Should Take to Help Me Lose Weight?

The short answer to that is no, there are no supplements that you have to take in order to lose weight. Are there supplements out there that could give you a little boost? Yes.

Are they worth it? Probably not.

Companies that want your money have really overhyped supplements. They market their products to make it seem as if all you have to do is take this pill without doing anything else and boom you'll lose weight.

Deep down, we know it's not that easy, but we want it to be true so badly that we try it anyway. And that's why supplements companies make so much money.

They prey on people who aren't willing to do the hard (but necessary) stuff and who want the easy way out. I'm here to tell you that there is no easy way out.

You must follow sound nutrition and/or exercise principles in order to obtain your desired fitness result. I think you're better off skipping supplements and focusing on your diet plan as your main way of losing weight.

This isn't what supplement companies want you to hear, but it's the truth. Not only that, but think about what the word supplement means.

It's meant to supplement something (a sound diet or exercise plan in this case) not be a total replacement for it. Yet many people look to these supplements as magic, and they certainly are nothing of the sort.

With that being said, if you had some extra money on hand and there's a supplement you really want to try out, you certainly can. Just be cautious that you never buy a supplement with the expectations that it'll do all of the hard work for you because it certainly won't.

Conclusion

The military diet will certainly toughen you up and help you lose weight. The main thing is to be diligent but to also have patience. If you have a lot of weight to lose, you're not going to hit your goal overnight. You must have the patience to see things through until the end. If you're able to do that, then not only will you lose weight, but you'll be able to keep it off.

Sources

(1) https://www.cdc.gov/nchs/fastats/obesity-overweight.htm

(2) https://www.ncbi.nlm.nih.gov/pubmed/16579728

(3) https://www.ncbi.nlm.nih.gov/pubmed/7369170

(4) https://www.ncbi.nlm.nih.gov/pmc/articles/PMC4391809/

(5) https://www.ncbi.nlm.nih.gov/pmc/articles/PMC3289193/

(6) https://www.ncbi.nlm.nih.gov/pubmed/15518309

(7) https://www.mayomedicallaboratories.com/test-catalog/Clinical+and+Interpretive/83686

(8) http://www.ncbi.nlm.nih.gov/pubmed/18197184

(9) http://www.ncbi.nlm.nih.gov/pubmed/20473222

(10) https://www.ncbi.nlm.nih.gov/pmc/articles/PMC1470658/

(11) https://www.ncbi.nlm.nih.gov/pmc/articles/PMC2782938/